CBD Hemp Oil

The Complete Guide To Using CBD Oil For Health, Pain Relief, Anxiety And Overall Wellness

TY GODSON

DEDICATION

For Grandma, Belle

Loving memories always!

TABLE OF CONTENT

INTRODUCTION

Chronic pain, muscle pain, arthritis, migraines, spinal cord injuries or muscle spasms; no type of pain is easy to live with. Anxiety, seizures, psychosis, insomnia, neurodegenerative disorders, acne and many others, are conditions that a large number of people constantly face and seek solutions to. It is imperative that they do; you can't have a pleasant and fulfilling day when you're battling pain, neither can you be productive to yourself, your family and society at large when your health is failing. When you have tried modern medicine and symptoms persist, it is advisable to go in search of natural remedies, especially in the form of CBD.

In recent times, CBD has become a very popular mode of addressing pain. It is generally used by patients in the form of oil. Hundreds of reviewed studies show that CBD oils have remarkable clinical potentials. There have been incredible stories of how CBD has transformed lives. Studies have shown that CBD oil is extremely effective for pain alleviation, and is a safe alternative to opiods. Opiods are powerful drugs that are used to treat acute pain. However, it is commonly abused. It is reported that more than a hundred Americans die from opiod overdose every day! CBD has no risk of abuse. The effectiveness of CBD treatment for pain is mind-blowing, so much so, that even doctors are now recommending it in place of traditional pain treatments. CBD users, who made the switch from prescription pain killers, also attest to its safety and efficacy.

Side effects such as sleep disruptions, digestive issues, irritability and suicidal thoughts that come with using pharmaceuticals are now a thing of the past. Why? CBD has no side-effects. According to the World Health Organization (WHO), CBD is not only safe and well tolerated; it is also "not associated with any significant adverse public health effects." Virtually every test on CBD's effectiveness produced positive effects. The only negative side effect that was obtained was caused by using too much CBD, and the effect was just a slight fatigue. CBD also supports general health and well-being. Consequently, it can be taken by every one! The only restriction that may occur may be for medical or health reasons. This is why it is always advisable to seek the counsel of a medical professional before usage, especially if you are taking regular prescription medicines.

CBD is redefining natural heath and healing. With it, you can restore your health, revitalize your body and remain healthy with minimal effort. It is extremely healthy and works wonders in treating a wide range of maladies and illnesses. This is not a fad or trend that will just come and go; the benefits of CBD had been widely confirmed and vigorously tested. So, you can put it to work and go to sleep!

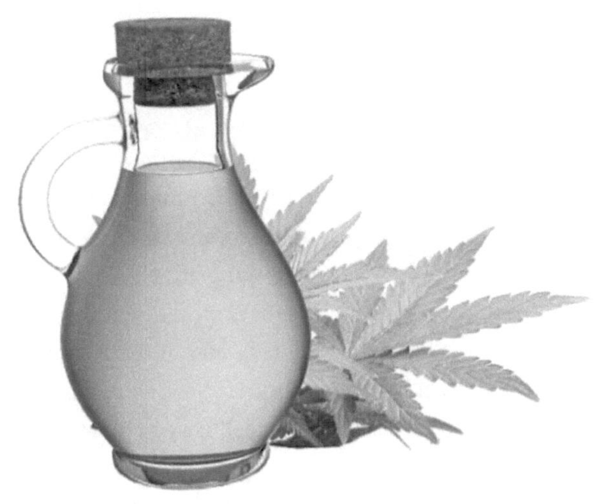

Understanding CBD & THC

CBD, short for cannabidiol, is an active chemical compound, called cannabinoid, which is found in the plants of the cannabis family and proven to possess tremendous health benefits. There are more than a hundred cannabinoids in the cannabis plant. Cannabidiol (CBD) is just one of them while tetrahydrocannabinol (THC) is another. These two are the most popular cannabinoid, the most studied and the most documented. However, THC is the most abundant cannabinoid in the cannabis plant; while CBD is the second. CBD and THC may come from the same plant, but they are not the same. CBD and THC are two completely separate cannabinoids. THC is a psychoactive compound, while CBD is non-psychoactive. This means CBD will not get you high or stoned.

CBD is naturally calming and soothing. Unlike TCH, CBD will enable you go about your daily task, like working, commuting, driving and looking after your children without any risks. Your senses won't be dulled and normal faculties will be intact. This is one of the reasons why CBD can offer relief from inflammation, pain, anxiety, seizures, spasms, psychosis without feelings of lethargy. CBD can relieve myriad diseases. It is great for spasm. It reduces the symptoms affecting the body and the overall quality of life and it does this without triggering any unwanted side effects like THC. With CBD is all relaxation, with no intoxication.

Although Marijuana is part of the cannabis family, it does not work like CBD because it contains a different type of cannabinoid, known as THC. THC is the psychoactive compound in marijuana that gives user the high feeling. Marijuana products are usually made from cannabis plants that are highly concentrated with THC. On the average, a batch of marijuana can have between 5-20% THC contents. Some premium marijuana can even have as much as 25-30% THC.

THC is not altogether 'bad'. It can help alleviate the side effects of chemotherapy, glaucoma and multiple sclerosis. But CBD performs exceedingly better, and without side effects! With CBD, you can lessen anxiety and paranoia, treat inflammation, and much more. It is important to point out that certain marijuana strains are rich in CBD. This is because marijuana cultivators have found a way to create strains that have very high levels of CBD. An example of a very popular one is Charlotte's Web. There are many others in the market.

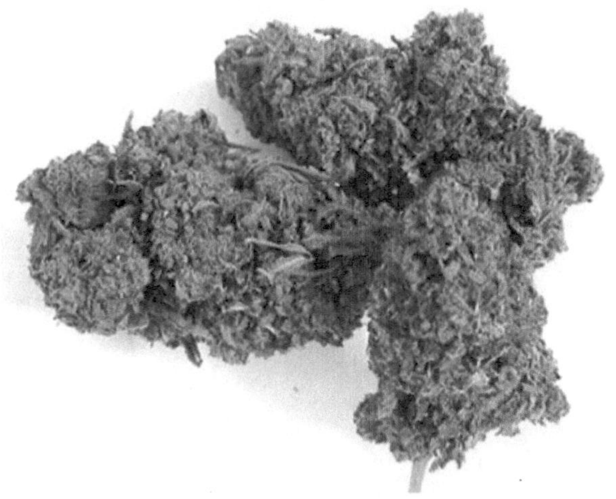

Hemp, from which CBD is generally extracted and separated, contains only a maximum THC level of 0.3%. But it contains high cannabidiol (CBD), up to 40% that helps to counter the adverse effect of THC. The remaining 60% contains many other compounds.

CBD as a term generally refers to cannabis plant extract that is high in Cannabidiol with smaller amounts of other compounds. These other compounds include cannabigerol (CBG), cannabichromene (CBC) and cannabinol (CBN) as well as terpenes, vitamins, amino acids, fatty acids and trace minerals. Most companies that produce CBD oil extract it from hemp, leaves, stalks, and flowers. The extraction method is called CO2.

Understanding Cannabis, Hemp & Marijuana

<u>Cannabis</u>

Cannabis is one of the oldest domesticated crops. For thousands of years, this plant has been used for its medicinal value. This is on account of its inflammatory, sedative/hypnotic, antidepressant, and anticonvulsant properties as well as its anti-spasmodic, analgesic and appetite-stimulating properties. Different varieties of the cannabis plant were also grown for their industrial benefits as well as for recreation; an example of this is the industrial hemp and marijuana. Industrial hemp was grown to produce fibers, while marijuana was used for recreational purposes.

The name cannabis is not really synonymous with marijuana; it is simply the genus or general umbrella term which all kinds of marijuana and hemp fall under. There are three different growing varieties or species of cannabis (cannabis genus):

1. Cannabis Savita: This is the most common strain of cannabis. It has been cultivated since the beginning of time for foods, oils, fabrics and ropes. It is even cultivated for recreation. This specie contains higher levels of THC over CBD. CBD compound is found in the cannabis Sativa.

2. Cannabis Indica: This specie is shorter and bushier than Sativa. It contains higher levels of CBD over THC, and lastly,

3. Cannabis Ruderalis: This strain has the ability to endure harsher conditions than the others. It contains only low levels of THC. This THC level is the lowest of the three.

The different properties and strains of the cannabis plant were cultivated for different purposes: For instance,

1. Industrial hemp is grown from Sativa to produce minimal levels of THC that are used in producing hemp oil, resin, wax, hemp seed, animal feed, cloth, fuel, rope, and many others.

2. Medical marijuana is grown solely to maximize Cannabinoid concentration, while

3. Ruderalis is exclusively cultivated because of its very small quantities of THC.

Many different strains have since been developed from these original three. This is why the THC level of a plant is often used to correctly determine its status; rather than strictly labeling them as Sativa or Indica.

Hemp & Marijuana

Hemp and marijuana come from the same plant (cannabis). Therefore, hemp and marijuana are different varieties or species of the cannabis plant. Industrial hemp is solely by the Cannabis Sativa, but marijuana can be cultivated from the Cannabis Sativa, Cannabis Indica, or Cannabis Ruderalis. Hemp and marijuana are specific part of the plant. Hemp refers to the sterilized stems, stalks, seeds and roots. Marijuana refers to the viable seeds, leaves and flowers of the plant, which contains the highest THC levels

Nevertheless, the major difference between industrial hemp and medical marijuana is the way they are bred. Hemp-producing Cannabis is fibrous and strong with tall stalks and a handful of flowering buds. On the contrary, marijuana strains of cannabis are short, with many flowering buds as possible, and contain high amounts of THC. Marijuana is bred with the sole purpose of maximizing the concentration of THC, but industrial hemp is specifically bred to produce the lowest possible concentrations of THC.

Industrial hemp naturally has trace amounts of THC and fairly high quantities of CBD. It is chemically impossible for it to induce intoxicating effects. Hemp is a very versatile and high-growing plant. Therefore, it is used to create medicines, food and oil as well as other products such as rope, natural polymers, fiber and bricks. People who want to benefit from cannabis without the high effect often find the cannanbidol profile of hemp ideal for their situations.

Marijuana has a high amount of THC and very low amount of CBD. It is exclusively for recreational and medicinal use. Each strain of marijuana is on a ratio of THC-to-CBD spectrum. Some marijuana has higher levels of THC and lower amounts of CBD. For others, it is vice-versa. Patients who wish to use both CBD and THC to address their symptoms go for high-CBD marijuana strains, whereas patients who are interested only in the non-psychoactive properties of CBD favor high-CBD hemp oil.

Note that CBD oil is cannabis oil, irrespective of whether it is derived from industrial hemp or marijuana. This is as long as it has a considerable amount of cannabidiol in it. CBD products that are extracted and derived from industrial hemp are considered or referred to as CBD hemp oil. They can also be known as hemp-derived CBD oil or CBD- rich cannabis oil. Some oil that contain more than CBD are considered hemp extracts. To reiterate, CBD hemp, with low amounts of THC, cannot get you

high. Its oil contains no THC so they cannot get you high,
you can't get any disjointed feeling, nor will you feel
lethargic.

The Many Benefits Of CBD Oil

1. For Pain Relief

CBD-rich cannabis has a documented history of acting as a remedy for pain. In the mid 19th century, UK Queen, Queen Victoria, used CBD to alleviate her menstrual cramps. A 2011 fibromyalgia study also indicated results. Of the 112 participants of the study, 56 of those who took CBD treatment showed significant reduction of their pain and symptoms compared to those who took the traditional methods. CBD oil is effective for pain management due to its effects on the brain receptors. Studies have also proven its pain relieving benefits for chemotherapy. It alleviates pain brought about by arthritis, muscle pain, MS pain, and spinal cord injuries.

2. For Anxiety Relief

CBD will help you manage anxiety. It is known to aid relaxation. Anxiety disorders are a group of mental illnesses that can disrupt day-to-day function. People with anxiety disorders usually have fears and worries that are overwhelming and disabling. When we consume CBD oil, it makes changes to our brain receptors, known as CB1. The cells in our brain respond to chemical signals from different stimuli. CBD alters serotonin signals. Serotonin is a chemical that plays a role in our mental health. Too little of it affects mental health. CBD provides relief from post- traumatic stress (PTSD), Seasonal Affective Disorder (SAD) social anxiety disorder and anxiety- induced insonmia. Cannabidiol also relives the anxiety sufferer by reducing the stress and decreasing heart rate that is usually associated with public speaking.

3. For Seizures

Worldwide, about 50 million people live with epilepsy. Epilepsy is a neurological condition that involves frequent seizures. Epilepsy makes life very difficult for the sufferers. Simple tasks like driving, preparing food, caring for children and keeping a job or career become overwhelming. The sufferers also experience depression and anxiety. Epileptic seizures are caused by irregular electric misfiring or discharge among the brain cells. CBD, with its anticonvulsant properties, has been proven to reduce seizures in people with epilepsy by working on different targets in the brain.

In 2016, a study was conducted with 214 people suffering from epilepsy. Besides the existing medications they were taking to treat epilepsy, oral doses of 2-5mg of CBD were added to their daily doses. After 1 weeks of intense monitoring, checking the frequency of their seizures as well as noting any side effects, the study researchers noted that the seizures reduced by 36.5 percent within a month. Only 12 % of the participants had negative side effects.

For Neuro-Protection

CBD is a neuroprotectant. This means it has the ability to reduce damage to the brain and to the nervous system. It can help people with neurodegenerative disorders. Therefore people with Alzheimer's disease, stroke, Parkinson's disease and multiple sclerosis (MS) have a better chance of treatment with CBD. CBD oil also helps to reduce the inflammation that could worsen neurodegenerative. Research on CBD oil for neurodegenerative diseases is still ongoing.

For Cancer Treatment

According to the National Cancer Institute, CBD may prevent cancer cell growth. It can also lessen cancer symptoms and side effects caused by cancer treatments. Researchers think that since CBD can moderate inflammation and alter the way cell reproduce, it can reduce the ability of certain tumor cells to reproduce. Research for this, however, is still in its primary stages.

For Curbing Cigarette Addiction

Studies also show that CBD can curb cigarette addiction. 24 smokers were placed on either a CBD inhaler or placebo. After one week, those with placebo inhalers still smoked the same number of cigarettes that they usually smoke; while those placed on inhalers with CBD had their addiction reduced by 40%.

For Treating Crohn's Disease

CBD can help with bowel diseases like Crohn's Disease. CBD anti-inflammatory properties make it possible for it to alleviate the symptoms of Crohn's disease, bringing lasting relief to the sufferers. These symptoms include: abdominal pain, fatigue, joints and muscles' soreness as well as intestinal inflammation. It also stimulates appetite which prevents weight loss and leads to proper weight gain, and it does all these without causing withdrawal symptoms unlike other pharmaceutical drugs for bowel diseases.

For Beauty

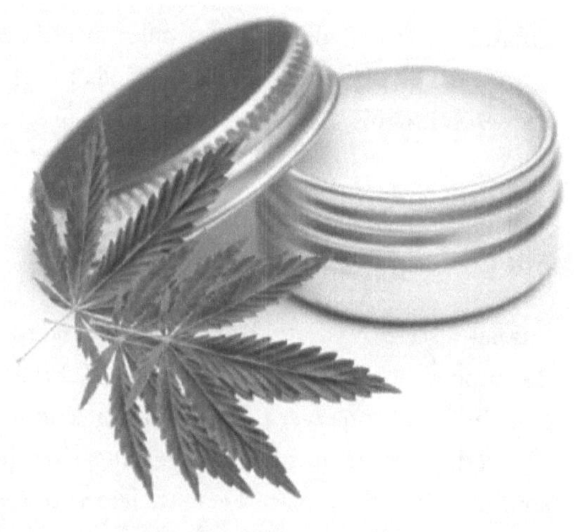

CBD oil is effective for treating acne. It moisturizes and soothes the skin. It also helps the skin to retain moisture. Since CBD oil is rich fatty acids, it fill in the cracks between skin cells, eliminating dry skin and treating issues like acne and eczema. Many cosmetics companies have begun to add CBD to their ingredients list.

Benefits of CBD oil

In a nutshell, CBD Oil:

- Reduces nausea and vomiting: gastro-intestinal disorders usually bring about such symptoms like nausea and vomiting. This is where CBD oil can help. Additionally, it can be used to address the discomfort and pain that comes from chemotherapy and radiotherapy treatments for malignant tumors.

- If you're battling cancer, CBD oil may increase your body's capacity to fight the cells accusing it and make your life better while undergoing treatments.

- Helps with all kinds of seizures

- Helps you quit smoking

- Helps with insomnia

- Helps with Schizophrenia

- Helps the immune system

- Promotes bone growth

- Reduces Blood Sugar

- Reduces Anxiety

- Provides treatment for acne

- Helps to reverse type11 diabetes and manage type 1 diabetes.

- Alleviate Parkinson, Alzheimer, and other neuro-generative disorders

- Reduces joint aches

- Alleviates fibromyalgia

- Great in alleviating PTSD by reducing its debilitating symptoms and increasing quality of life.

Why CBD Oil Works So Well

The human brain is extremely complex. It is also a very important organ that interacts with all other organs in our body as well as interacts with innumerable physiological and psychological processes. As a matter of fact, our health and happiness depends on the functionality of this great organ.

Cannabinoids affect our brain and central nervous system, the endocannabinoid system (ECS), by activating their receptors. ECS is the largest neurotransmitter network in the human body. ECS is important because it regulates mood, appetite, memory, pain, inflammation and aging. It also plays important roles in the immune, cardiovascular, reproductive, and gastrointestinal systems. By far, the most important work of the ECS is to regulate the stability of all the functions of the body. This is known as homeotatsis. ECS is involved in numerous areas of our health. Consequently, it helps to restore balance when we are ill or make poor diet choices.

So how does Cannabinoids activate ECS receptors? Our body has naturally-occurring cannabinoid cell receptors which control processes like thought, pain and immune system. These receptors also act as keyholes to chemicals produced in the human body. These chemicals include THC, CBN and cannabidiol, (female breast milk contains cannabidiol). In the human body, there are two types of cannabinoid receptors found on cell surfaces:

CBD 1 receptors are concentrated in brain, central nervous systems and nerves.

CBD 2 receptors are mostly found in peripheral organs, especially cells that are linked with the immune system.

Therefore, when any of these two cannabinoids, THC and CBD interact with our cannabinoid receptors, they respond in different ways. CBD, on its own part, affects so many of our bodily processes. It also brings about physical and mental changes without causing side effects. It does all these because of our biochemistry. CBD helps to modulate many physiological systems in the human brain and body.

CBD oil contains active, biochemical ingredients that make it great for healing. The alkaloids (the active substances in CBD oil) make it possible for it to lower overall inflammation in the body and stimulate the parasympathetic nervous system. This triggers the body to enter into its rejuvenation or recovery mode. CBD is safe to use because it interacts naturally with our system.

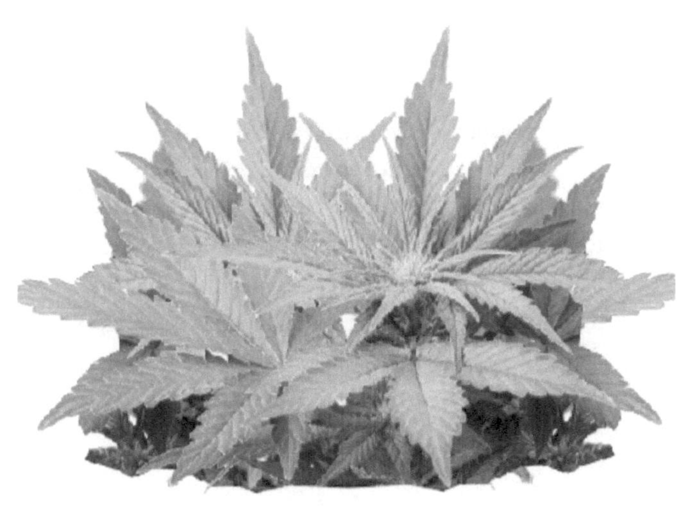

How To Use CBD Oils

As mentioned earlier, CBD is extracted from the hemp plant in oil or powder form. The oil or powder can be mixed into creams or gels. They can be put in capsule form and ingested. They can also be applied topically. Nabiximols, is a multiple sclerosis drug that is sprayed into the mouth as a liquid. To a large extent, the usage of CBD depends on what the user wants to use it for. Be sure to consult your doctor before using CBD oil.

CBD products are available in various forms:

1. <u>CBD Oils:</u> This is the most powerful type of CBD product available. CBD oil is extracted from the hemp plant and used with no addictives. They are pure and highly concentrated. However, they are very expensive.

2. <u>CBD Capsules:</u> Taking CBD oil in capsule form is a great way of getting CBD into your daily routine. CBD capsules usually contain about 25 mg of CBD.

3. <u>CBD Tinctures or Liquids:</u> CBD oil products are also available in liquid forms. It is produced by diluting CBD oil into an alcohol or any other natural oil base. It is also known as CBD tinctures or sprays. One benefit of using CBD in this form is that they come in very small serving; between 1-20 mg, which is manageable, adequate and

convenient for most people. The most beneficial advantage of CBD tinctures, liquids or sprays is its affordability. They are the most affordable products available.

4. <u>CBD Topicals:</u> Besides using CBD internally, it can also be used topically. CBD oils are mixed into salves and balms and applied directly on the skin. Most CBD topicals contain other all-natural ingredients like essential oils that are blended and rubbed to trouble areas of the skin, muscles and joints. This helps to address many skin ailments such as acne, eczema and rough skin as well as many other skin ailments that are caused by inflammation.

By applying CBD oils topically, you can be sure of a relatively slow but even absorption. Your skin will remain moisturized and enjoy CBD's benefits for a much longer period of time. For pain relief, CBD oil can also be applied locally, for instance, on the forehead to eliminate tension headaches.

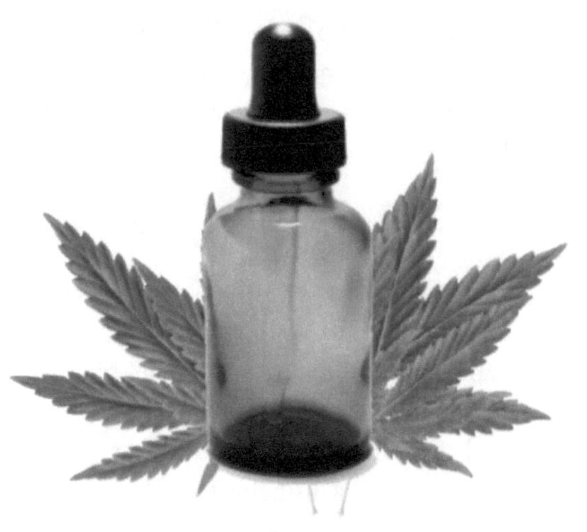

For Kids...

CBD oil is safe for children. As a matter of fact, you can treat several childhood illnesses and conditions, particularly epilepsy with CBD oil. It is not just safe; but safer than common medications, such as aspirin. CBD oil is available in a range of great flavors. Children with a sweet tooth will also benefit from these flavors.

And Pets

CBD is safe for dogs, cats, and other animals. Numerous studies have been conducted on animals and none of these studies have brought out adverse results. This indicates that CBD oil is safe to use for animals.

CBD for pets addresses health issues like joint pain, epilepsy, anxiety and skin problems.

There are pre-made CBD dog treats that you can buy for your dog. Be sure to get them from a reputable company. Check the label. The CBD oils you buy must list the amount of CBD that is in each drop, otherwise, do not buy it, or use. Reputable companies measure this amount in milligrams (mg). The label should also indicate the number of drops to give your dog.

Below is the general recommendation for smaller dogs

10 lbs: 1-5 mg

20 lbs: 2-10 mg

30 lbs: 3-15 mg

If there are no noticeable changes within an hour, the dosage can be increased. It is advisable to find what suits your dog. It is always safe to begin with the lowest recommended dose, and then increase it a little at a time.

Dosages

Dosages vary from person to person. Everybody reacts differently to CBD oils. The tolerance level of the individual must be put into consideration. Some people are very sensitive and will need just little. There are also rare cases of people who won't feel the effect even after taking powerful dosages.

Although CBD oils are easy to take, it doesn't taste well. Nevertheless, you must hold it under your tongue for a minute or two before swallowing. This will enable it to absorb through your mucus membrane instead of your stomach. This route is much more effective. You only need a few drops under your tongue and it goes immediately into your system. A lot of people gradually reduce the amount of CBD taken once they have built in into their system.

For CBD oil, the recommended dose is:

- A tiny drop of oil under the tongue, three times daily during the first week of use.
- For the second week, double the dosage by applying 2 drops under your tongue.
- If you like, you can double the dosage every 4-7 days until the maximum dosage of 300mg/ml daily (21 to 24 drops in a syringe = 1 ml) is attained after 6-8 weeks.

Keep at this dose, not adding to it, until the ailment disappears. Once you build your dosage up to the maximum level of 1ml a day, you will develop body tolerance. After maintaining this regimen for 3-6 months, you will be able to maintain your health with just one drop of CBD oil twice a day.

Note that more concentrated the CBD oil is; the better. For faster effect, it is best to take CBD oil on an empty stomach. The strength of the effect depends on how much of a dosage you take and the symptoms you want to tackle. Additionally, bear in mind that CBD is not water soluble. What this means is that it will not mix with water or juice. So if you add your CBD oil to your drink, you have to wait much longer, between 20 minutes to an hour for the effects to become noticeable. It is also advisable to take CBD oil in moderation, even if they aren't much research concerning overconsumption of CBD, except a few complaints of stomach discomfort and fatigue.

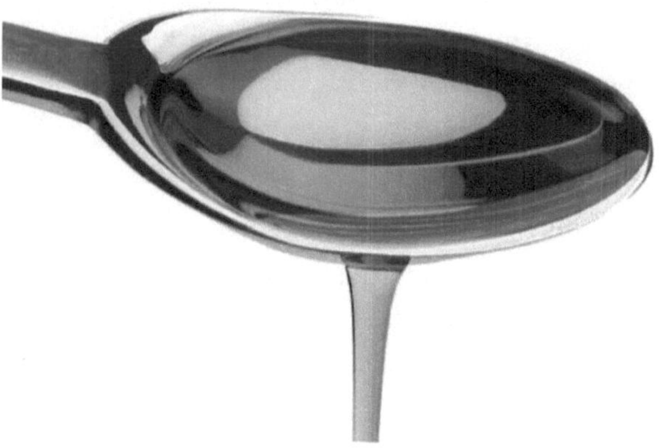

You can buy CBD oil from any reputable producer. You do not need a permit or a doctor's recommendation to buy one. You can even make yours. But remember that you must always start with low dosages; then you can slowly increase it. But, if you have chronic illness and take some medication, it is imperative you inform your physician before you start taking CBD. And in the rare event your symptoms worsen, lower your dose or stop using completely.

The Legality Of CBD

CBD products produced from industrial hemp are legal in any state. As long as CBD is produced through the proper means, it is legal everywhere. Additionally, since CBD oil does not contain the psychoactive properties of THC, it is legal. Nevertheless, some cannabis-infused skincare and health products can only be bought in states where marijuana is already legal.

In the USA, it is illegal to grow your own hemp and process it into CBD. You can only do so if have obtained proper licenses and permits. For this reason, most CBD oil is imported. It is difficult to control and regulate. This is one very important reason you must be cautious of the brand that you buy and carry out a due diligence before purchase.

DO IT-YOURSELF RECIPES

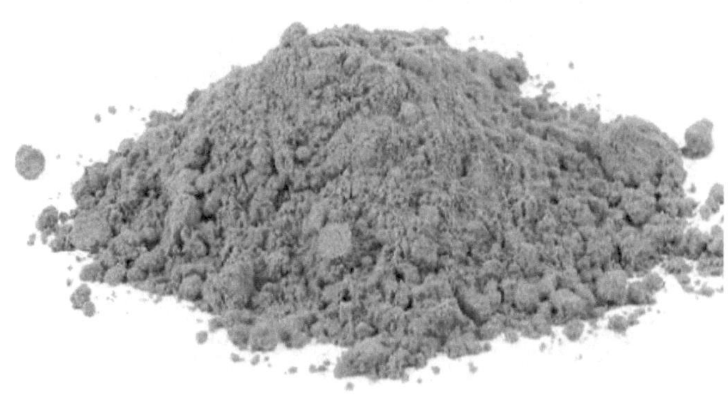

Make Your Own CBD Oil

Making your own CBD oil will save you up to 50% on cost. It may even be of a higher quality than those in the market. Some unscrupulous companies can decide to add chemical addictives in their oils. But when you make yours, you control what goes into it. There are many ways to make CBD oil. Let's consider a few:

Potent CBD Oil

This is a very potent CBD oil mix made with grain alcohol, because it is the best. It leaves no harmful residues in the extraction. Additionally, it is safe and just suitable for creating small homemade batches of CBD oil.

Ingredients

30g of ground buds

4L of grain alcohol, high-proof alcohol

Equipment

Double boiler

Mixing bowl, ceramic or glass

Electric stove

Wooden spoon

Mason jar

Cheesecloth or sieve

Silicon spatula

Catchment container

Funnel

Plastic syringe

Instructions

1. Place the cannabis in a mixing bowl. Pour over the alcohol, stir and let it stay overnight.

2. Using the cheesecloth or sieve, filter the raw extraction into a container.

3. Pour the extracted liquid into a double boiler and then heat at very low until bubbles start to form

4. Let the alcohol evaporate completely; and ensure the heat is set at very low. You may turn it off and on to regulate the temperature.

5. Let the mixture keep bubbling for about 30 minutes. Do not let the mixture get too hot! Continue to stir to let in some air.

6. Mix the solution with a silicon spatula and scrape bowl.

6. Transfer the concentrated oil gently into a storage bottle. Do not wait for it to cool; otherwise, it'll get too thick

7. Draw the CBD oil with a plastic syringe and then remove to a small dark, airtight container.

Note: Natural CBD extracts are usually thick and concentrated. However, they can be diluted with any vegetable oil, such as olive oil or coconut oil upon completion of the process.

Coconut CBD Oil

Ingredients

1 gram CBD isolate

1 cup coconut oil

Instructions

1. Grind the CBD isolate to powder and place in a pot.

2. Add the coconut oil

3. Simmer on lowest temperature and stir to dissolve CBD completely

4. Pour into a glass jar

Note: This will give you 48 teaspoons of coconut CBD oil at 20mg of CBD in one serving. Shelf life is at least 2 months.

CBD Hemp Oil For Topical Use

Ingredients

1 cup Extra Virgin Coconut Oil

14g organic hemp CBD buds and leaves

Instructions

1. Grind the buds of the hemp plant as well as its stems and leaves; you can do this with a coffee grinder.

2. Transfer hemp to a small glass jar, pour the oil over it and seal tightly.

3. Place a wash rag in a small pan and then place the jar in the pan. Pour 2-3 inches of water in the pan and bring the water to boiling; set at 180 degrees

4. Heat water this way for 3-4 hours and add more water so it doesn't dry out. Shake the jar carefully after every hour.

5. Now turn off heat, cover pot with a towel and let the jar remain in there for another 3-6 hours. Leave the jar in there overnight.

6. Repeat this process for the next 3 days if possible. (While it can be used after one day, the oil will be stronger if it sits longer, at least 3 days).

7. Now strain oil and herbs into another jar, with the help of a cheesecloth.

8. Use oil topically

CBD Tinctures

CBD tinctures are liquid solutions that blend CBD oil with ethanol, glycerin or other type of nutritious oil. Most people find CBD tinctures simple and convenient, it is considered as a versatile way of getting your daily dose of CBD. Most tinctures contain a very strong concentration of 10% to 25% CBD. Tinctures can be made with alcohol or glycerin. You can buy CBD tinctures online or make your own.

Alcohol/ Ethanol Tincture

1/2 g CBD isolate or 2 g CBD hemp oil

1½ tbsp MCT oil or coconut oil

Equipment

1-ounce dropper bottle

Small funnel

Instruction

1. Get a double boiler, pour 1 to 2 inches water in the bottom pan and place on the stove. Set heat to low.

2. Place the upper pan of the double boiler onto the bottom one and then add the MCT oil and the CBD Isolate powder, stirring gently to dissolve.

3. Remove double boiler from heat. Cool CBD tincture.

4. Using a funnel, pour CBD tincture from the pan into the dropper bottle. Chill.

Or Alcohol-Free CBD- Glycerin Tincture

A glycerin tincture is affordable and safe. Since it is alcohol free, it is suitable for all. It's also completing customizable, enabling you to select the strains that you desire.

Ingredients

1 oz your high-CBD flower shake & nugs

Vegetable glycerin

Instructions

1. Grind CBD flower shake into fine powder

2. Add the glycerin and transfer to a mason jar, sealing tightly.

3. Place jars on a window sill for maximum exposure to sunlight and let it sit for 6-7 weeks to marinate, shaking once in a day to activate the cannabinoids.

4. Remove the extracted cannabis by straining the tincture through a cheesecloth or cheese.

5. Pour the tincture into a dropper bottle and chill.

Making CBD-infused ingredients

CBD oils can be added to ingredients that you want to cook with. Here are common ways to do this:

CBD Oil-Infused Butter

Butter is a versatile ingredient that can be added to many tasty snacks. However, the CBD oil must slowly be infused into the butter and over a low heat. This will incorporate the CBD without getting it scorched, and without evaporating the active compounds.

Ingredients

500g butter

15 ml of CBD oil

Instructions

1. To begin, cut the butter into pieces, and then place the pieces in a medium saucepan. Pour in the CBD oil, and a quart of water.

2. Set the heat on low, and cook for 3 to 4 hours. Check it often and stir every 30 minutes.

3. Once the CBD oil and butter is well combined, pour mixture into a bowl, and refrigerate for 2hours.

Note

Enjoy over some hot popcorn by melting the butter, as condiment on meat or potatoes, to make biscuits, or as spread on toast. Or any favorite baked goods that you like.

CBD-Infused Oils

If you don't like butter, you can still make a versatile CBD-infused oil for use in several recipes. CBD oil is fat soluble. It can be added to any fat. Coconut oil and olive oil work very well in this regard. Coconut oil in particular, is popularly used because it is easier to digest and safer to use even in high temperature. Simply use the same method for infusing butter to infuse any of these oils. Once made, these CBD-infused oils can be used in lots of ways. A few of these includes sautéing vegetables and garlic or for deep frying, or to make homemade granola bars, potato chips or vegetable chips like beets or carrots.

CBD Smoothies

Drinking a smoothie as a meal, particularly breakfast, has become a healthy trend. Packed full of nutrients, smoothies that includes CBD oil is a great way to start the day. It will take away any aches or pains that you might have had when you wake and will also eliminate any anxieties you may have. CBD oil does not affect the texture of the drink. It is also a healthy dessert choice in the course of your day, instead of the traditional sugary ice cream.

CBD Oils To Pastas

Pasta is a very popular CBD-infused edible. CBD can be incorporated into savory pasta dishes by putting the oil in creamy or cheesy dishes. Baked Mac and cheese and lasagna are good examples. But remember that it shouldn't be baked at high temperatures. It is always better to add CBD oil a little at a time, so that you won't overdo it. Then next time, you can be sure of the exact CBD oil to incorporate.

CBD-Infused Salad Dressings/ Condiment

The safest way of using CBD oil is to add it to salad dressings and other conditions. This way, you won't overcook the oil. Your CBD-infused oil can be used to make a vinaigrette salad dressing. In addition, it can be used as marinade for your meats or fish as well as add to shelf-stable condiments like barbecue sauce and ketchup.

To use CBD-infused butter:

- Top your popcorn, toast or potatoes
- Add to your favorite brownie or cookie

To use CBD-infused oil:

- Add to salad dressings and sauces
- Add to pasta
- Sauté vegetables
- Roast vegetables

- Make oven-baked vegetable chips
- Add to spicy Thai curries to conceal the oil taste
- Use in smoothies
- Add to alcohol drinks by soaking in brandy, vodka, gin, or whiskey.
- Add to non-alcoholic drinks

CBD Edibles

Foods infused with CBD (Cannabidiol) are referred to as CBD edibles. They help to calm and relax the body and mind. Once you have purchased or made your CBD oil, there are so many ways you can infuse these very versatile substance to your meals, as pointed out earlier. There are a few things to note though:

1. Buy From A Reliable Source

There are lots of sellers of CBD oil; but they aren't all reliable. Also their products may not be pure, well tested, or correctly measured. Check through different brands, taking time to know vital information like the source of the hemp as well as the extraction methods.

2. CBD Is Fat Soluble

CBD is Fat Soluble. This is why butter or oil is the method that is most commonly used to craft cannabis infused edibles. Other fats that can be used for cannabidiol edibles include:

- Butter
- Olive Oil
- Coconut Oil
- Glycerin

3. Know Your Ingredients

Before you cook with CBD oil, you should consider all other ingredients that you want to use and the effect on the oil when combined. Thankfully, CBD is fat soluble and works well with butter or oil. But if you do not have those in your ingredient list, it is best you mix the oil with a little liquor like vodka or rum. But do not use any water-based one.

4. The Boiling Point Range

The boiling point range of Cannabidiol is between 160-180°C (320-356°F). Therefore, you must cook at low temperatures. Any temperature higher than the range given above may evaporate your CBD which will lower the effectiveness of your finished dish.

Since the oil begins to evaporate at 320 degrees, or thereabouts, when choosing a recipe, you must consider the temperature the food requires to be cooked at. This is essential for safe cooking and safe consumption and also to ensure that the CBD oil hasn't all evaporated after cooking. The lower the temperature, the more CBD you'll have in your food.

5. Be Moderate & Start With A Test Batch

Besides using a moderate amount of CBD oil, it is advisable to prepare a little quantity of the food you want to make. It is imperative that you check how the food tastes as well as if it has any effect on you. Once you've done this, then you can go ahead to use more oil in large amounts of food.

6. Calculate Serving Size Correctly

It is also important to calculate your serving size correctly so you can be sure of the exact CBD you are consuming in one serving. For instance, if a recipe says to use 4 tablespoons of your homemade CBD infused butter but instead you used an oil with 250mg of CBD, you will have to divide that particular number by the no. of servings you prepare so that you can have your serving Cannabidiol basis.

7. CBD is Heat & Light Sensitive

The heat and light sensitivity of CBD requires that you store it and other edibles correctly. If you don't, the taste might change or the oil may lose its potency or even evaporate. It should be stored in a cool dark place after use.

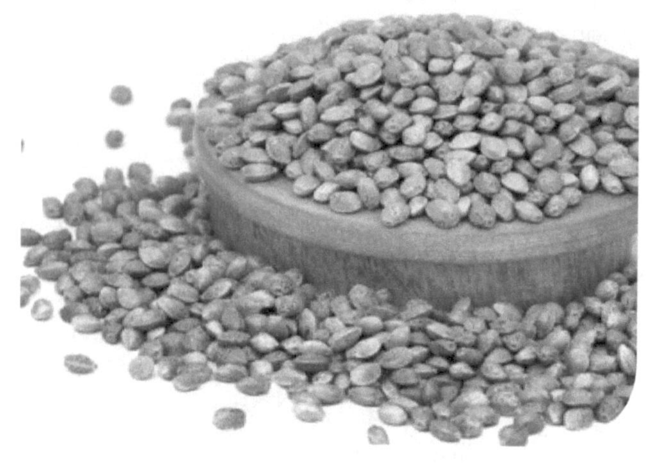

Homemade CBD Edibles

Enjoy crafting your own CBD edibles from home. It is safe, without side effects and versatile as well. The good thing about making your very own edibles is that you get to pick the exact amount of CBD oil or butter you desire in your food. There are so many tasty and healthy recipes to prepare with CBD.

Mac 'n Cheese

Serving Size: 4-6

Prep Time: 5 Minutes

Cook Time: 25-35 Minutes

Ingredients:

1/2 lb Elbow Macaroni

1 tbsp Canola Oil (Vegetable, Olive, or Coconut Oil)

1 tsp Salt

For the cheese sauce:

5 tbsp freshly made CBD Butter

1/2 to 3 Cups of Warm Milk

1/2 Cup of All-Purpose Flour

2 Cups of grated Cheddar

1 Cup of smoked cheese of choice

1 tsp kosher Salt

1 tsp Smoked Paprika

1/2 tsp Freshly Ground Black Pepper

1/2 tsp Ground Nutmeg

1 Cup Breadcrumbs

1 tbsp Canola oil , Optional

For the Onion Rings:

1 Small Onion, peeled and thinly sliced

1 Cup of Canola Oil (Or Oil of Your Choice)

Directions

1. Preheat oven to 375 Degrees F.

2. Add water to a large pot and then add oil and salt. Add the noodles and cook as directed on package.

3. Now place the cannabidiol butter in a small pan and melt on the stove, add flour, whisk often and cook 5 minutes.

4. Add milk and cook 1-2 minutes longer. Add the cheese sauce, paprika, nutmeg salt and pepper. Add the cooked macaroni and stir well. Transfer to a baking dish.

5. Combine breadcrumbs, sharp cheddar and canola oil in a small bowl. Sprinkle mixture over the macaroni that's in the baking dish. Bake for 25 to 35 minutes, until macaroni is golden brown on top and sauce is bubbly.

6. In a medium pan, heat the canola oil and once hot, add the sliced onion rings. Cook until golden brown, which is for about 5 minutes. Drain on paper towel and add to your Mac 'n cheese. Enjoy!

CBD-Infused Avocado Zinger Smoothie

Serving Size: 2

Approximate dosage: 5mg CBD per serving

Prep Time: 5 Minutes

Cook Time: 10 Minutes

Ingredients:

1 small, ripe banana, peeled & cut

10mg of CBD tincture

1½ cups coconut water

1 ripe avocado, halved and pitted

1½ tbsp lime juice

1 tablespoon Thai basil, chopped

1 teaspoon ginger, grated

1 cup of ice

Agave syrup, to taste (optional)

Directions

1. Scoop out flesh from avocado and place in the blender. Add the banana pieces and then the tincture drops, lime juice, coconut water, Thai basil, sugar and ginger.

2. Puree, add the ice and puree again until smooth.

3. Pour content into 2 glasses and add the agave syrup is desired.

CBD Milk

Fights insomnia and nighttime anxieties

Serving Size: 1

Prep Time: 5 Minutes

Cook Time: 0Minutes

Ingredients

2 cups hot water

1 1/2 tbsp coconut butter

1 tbsp tocos

40 milligrams CBD MCT oil

1 tsp Ceylon cinnamon

1 1/2 tsp ground ginger

1/2 tsp vanilla extract or 1 vanilla bean, insides scraped out

1/2 teaspoon reishi (optional)

Pinch pink salt

Directions

1. Add the hot water to a blender and then add the rest of the ingredients.

2. Blend on high 1-2 minutes until well-combined and frothy.

Cannbidiol Cakes Pancakes

Serving Size: 2-4

Prep Time: 20 Minutes

Cook Time: 20 Minutes

Ingredients:

1 1/4 Cups of Milk

1 Egg

1 1/4 Cups of Flour

2 Tablespoons of CBD Butter

2 Teaspoons of Sugar

2 Teaspoons of Baking Powder

1/4 Teaspoon of Salt

Optional ingredients:

Chocolate chips

Berries

Nuts

Fruits

Directions

1. In a large bowl, whisk together egg, milk and CBD butter until smooth.

2. In a separate bowl, combine flour, sugar, salt and baking powder and add to egg mixture, whisking until smooth.

3. Pour 1/3 cup batter onto a heated and oiled pan. Repeat for the rest of the batter. Cook pancake and flip once bubbles forms on it.

4. Enjoy!

Herbal Fudge Sundae

Serving Size:

Prep Time: 55 Minutes

Cook Time: 7Minutes

Ingredients

¼ cup cocoa

¼ cup whipping cream

¼ cup packed brown sugar

½ cup light corn syrup

8 oz semisweet chocolate bits

1 tbsp CBD butter

½ teaspoon pure vanilla extract

Directions

1, In a heavy saucepan, add the cocoa, whipping cream, sugar and corn syrup together. Melt over medium-low heat.

2. Remove pan, add the CBD butter and chocolate and stir frequently until thoroughly melted and smooth.

3. Now add the vanilla and stir once more. Scoop into dishes and top with desired sauce and toppings.

Infused Spinach Artichoke Dip

Ingredients:

2 cups parmesan cheese

10 oz frozen spinach

14 ounces artichoke hearts, drained &chopped

1 cup cream cheese

2/3 cup sour cream

1/3 cup mayonnaise

2 teaspoons garlic, minced

3 tablespoons CBD butter

Directions:

1. Add butter to pan, set on low heat and sauté the frozen spinach.

2. Now add parmesan cheese and artichoke hearts, missing to blend well.

3. Add sour cream, garlic, mayonnaise and cream cheese.

4. Serve hot with chips of choice, pita or Hawaiian bread.

CBD-Infused Mushroom Stew With Pasta

Serving Size: 4-6

Prep Time: 20 Minutes

Cook Time: 20Minutes

Ingredients

½ oz. dried shitake mushrooms

1 cup of hot water

4-6 tablespoons CBD-olive oil

2 leeks, rinsed& chopped

2 medium carrots, peeled & sliced

2 garlic cloves, peeled and sliced thinly

2 lbs. assorted mushrooms, cut evenly

2 tablespoons fresh rosemary, chopped

½ teaspoon salt

½ teaspoon pepper

16 oz. pasta of choice

Directions:

1. In a small bowl, add together the dried mushrooms and hot water. Let it sit 20 minutes.

2. Heat the olive oil in a large skillet; add the leeks and the carrots and sauté, 8 to 10 minutes until cooked. Add the garlic and mix well. Transfer content to a bowl.

3. Now add the fresh mushrooms to the pan and cook 8 to 10 minutes. Add the rosemary and the salt as well. Pour back the vegetables in the bowl to the pan, together with the soaked mushrooms and their liquid.

4. Cook pasta as instructed on package and divide among 6 plates. Place mushroom on top and enjoy warm.

Infused Breakfast Burrito

Ingredients:

2 tablespoons CBD oil

2 egg whites

2 spinach tortilla or whole wheat wraps

1/4 cup canned black beans, rinsed

1/4 cup cheese, fat free

Salsa (to taste)

Directions

1. Heat the CBD oil in pan.

2. Scramble the egg whites and cook.

3. Place the cooked eggs on heated tortilla and then sprinkle over cheese, beans and salsa.

4. Wrap together and enjoy!

Greens & Shrimp Pasta

Ingredients:

2 tablespoon CBD oil

3/4 lb angel hair pasta

1/4 tsp sea salt

2 tsp garlic, minced

1/4 tsp black pepper

1 pound raw medium shrimp peeled &deveined,

2 tbsp lemon zest, grated finely

3/4 cup heavy cream

10 oz baby spinach (about 12 cups), fresh or frozen

Directions

1. Cook pasta as directed on package; drain and place back in pot.

2. Rinse shrimp in cold water and then pat dry.

3. Melt CBD oil in a large skillet and then add the shrimp, salt, pepper and lemon zest, stirring often, between 4 to 5 minutes until the shrimp is opaque

4. Add the cream to pasta, cook over medium heat, stir and cook a minute or two or until slightly thickened, 1 to 2 minutes.

5. Add the shrimp mixture as well as the spinach and toss to combine.

CBD Oil Tomato Vinaigrette

Prep Time: 5 Minutes

Cook Time: 5Minutes

Ingredients

1 cup CBD-infused olive oil

1 cup cherry tomatoes

1/2 cup red wine vinegar

3 tbsp olive oil

1 tbsp Dijon mustard

2 teaspoons salt

1 teaspoon pepper

Directions

1. Sauté olive oil and tomatoes in a large pan.

2. Turn off heat, and bring to room temperature.

3. Transfer to blender; add the red wine vinegar and puree.

4. Add the mustard and drizzle over with CBD infused olive oil gently.

5. Season with salt and pepper.

Nut Butter Chocolaty Bars

Serving Size: 16

Prep Time: 15 Minutes

Cook Time: 25Minutes

Ingredients

1/2 cup vegetable oil canola

1/2 cup CBD infused vegetable oil

1/3 cup peanut butter

1 egg

1 cup brown sugar

1 cup all purpose flower

1 tsp vanilla extract

1 cup semi-sweet chocolate chips

Directions

1. Begin by preheating oven to 350 degrees and then grease baking pan.

2. Add the CBD-infused oil, vanilla extract, egg, brown sugar and peanut butter and whisk until smooth.

3. Now add flour and blend until well incorporate. Transfer to greased baking pan and spread evenly.

4. Add the chocolate chips and cook for 20 to 25 minutes in pre-heated oven.

5. Once done, cool on a wire rack; cut into bars and enjoy!

CBD Strawberry Sauce

Enjoy over a fruit salad, on top of your favorite dessert or mixed with white wine

Serving Size: 8

Prep Time: 20 Minutes

Cook Time: 45Minutes

Ingredients

2 tbsp. CBD Oil

1 lb. Strawberries, hulled & chopped finely

1/4 cup Honey

2 tsp. Cornstarch

1/2 cup Orange Juice, freshly squeezed

1 pinch Sea Salt

Directions

1. Add the strawberries, honey and CBD oil in a saucepan; set heat to medium-low and cook.

2. Combine cornstarch and orange juice in a small saucepan and add to the strawberries mixture on heat.

3. Stir and cook 8-10 minutes until sauce thickens.

4. Now remove, add salt and cool. Sauce will keep thickening as it cools.

The End